Hereditary Hemochromatosis? and Vitamin D Deficiency from UVB Radiation (sunlight) Originating from Northern Europe.

The Cause of Multiple Sclerosis

Hereditary Hemochromatosis? and Vitamin D Deficiency from UVB Radiation (sunlight) Originating from Northern Europe.

The Cause of Multiple Sclerosis

Trisha O'Connor

Rev. date: 05/15/2014

To order additional copies of this book, contact:
Xlibris LLC
1-888-795-4274
www.Xlibris.com
Orders@Xlibris.com
540250

Dedication

I dedicate the book to my son Connor Van Binnendÿk.
Also Grant Mackay for help with imaging and other computer
help for my book.
And my brother Kevin O'Connor for help with imaging.
Dr. Randall Phillips for continued medical support and help in
Byron in London Ontario.

ABSTRACT

In my survey 70% of MS patients had a Northern European ancestry consistent with the spread of the potato blight from 1845-1852. Iron Overload found in MS brains are from the mutated genes, C282Y,S65C and H63D from the HFE protein in the intestine in the 'cis' phase of hereditary hemochromatosis originating from Ireland.

Further genetic studies are needed for gender and age screening for hereditary hemochromatosis. MS patients will be deficient or have low levels vitamin B6, B12, or amino acids cysteine, taurine, glutathione, tyrosine, histidine, aspartic acid, lysine, methionine (reference 29), homocysteine or threonine, as well as defective enzymes for these amino acids.

Genes, Hereditary Hemochromatosis (HH), genetic screening, cysteine, tyrosine, and methionine.

Since 1989, the MS clinic in London, Ontario, Canada, has documented iron overload in brain autopsies of MS patients, indicating abnormalities in iron metabolism.[1] Then in 2008, Dr. P. Zamboni found blockages in the jugular and azygous veins in 90% of MS patients.[2] In 2009, Zamboni, et. al., stated genetic variation in gene coding for iron binding and transporting proteins could be accountable for the iron overload observed in a large number of MS patients.[2] Brain autopsies from the University Hospital in London, Ontario, Canada, throughout the 1980s have shown a substantial buildup of iron in patients with MS, which seems reasonable according to the research conducted by Zamboni regarding the changes in iron-related proteins in patients with

MS.[3] Then, in the late 1990s in Ferrara, Italy, Zamboni confirmed that there is indeed iron overload in the brains of MS patients.[2] Knowing that the mutated iron binding and transport genes, which were previously researched by Zamboni and led to iron overload, were also present in MS patients, we can state that MS patients are most likely of Irish and/or Northern European ancestry. We also know that 93% of Irish individuals who received treatment at a major hospital in Ireland were shown to have the mutated C282Y, S65C, and H63D on the HFE gene, which was used as a marker of hereditary hemochromatosis.[4]

What caused this mutated gene?

Could it be the Great Irish Potato Famine that caused this?

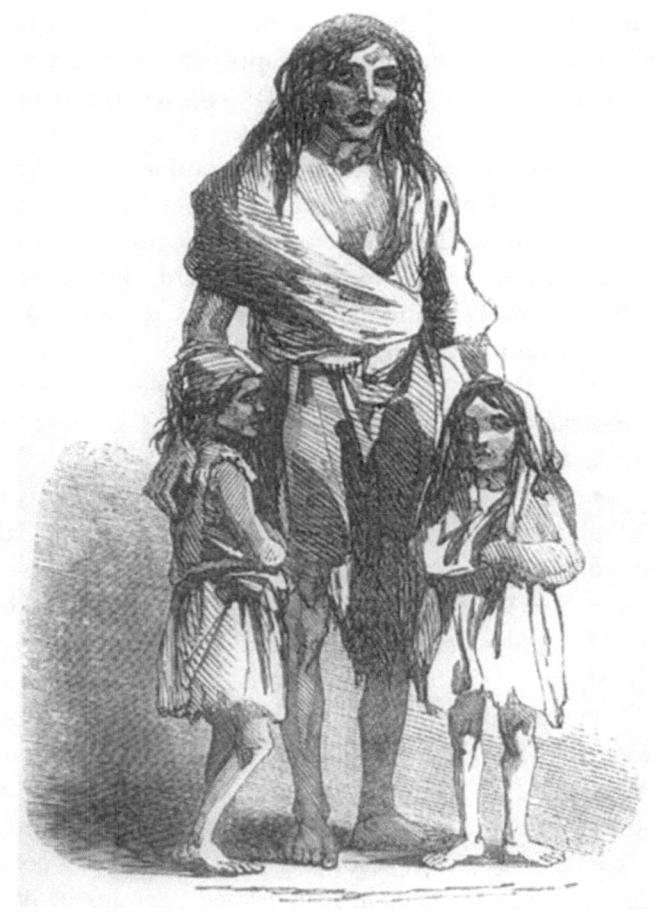

Between 1845 and 1852, the Great Irish Potato Famine was the worst disaster in the nineteenth century, killing one million and causing another two million to leave Ireland due to illness, accounting for about one-third of the country's population.[5] The potato blight spread quickly and by late summer / early autumn of 1845, it had already spread throughout the greater part of Northern and Central Europe, Belgium, Holland, Northern France, and Southern England, and by mid-August, the residents of these areas were already experiencing health concerns.[16] In 1844, the individuals who previously consumed the diseased potato immigrated overseas to the United States of America and the Great Lakes region in Canada, unknowingly bringing with them the associated health problems.[5]

The Great Irish Potato Famine that occurred in Ireland has yet to recover from the deaths and emigration from the mid nineteenth century.[26]

The potato crop had been infested by *Phytophthora infestans*, an oomycete—a type of single-celled organism related to brown algae, which caused the Irish potato blight.[26] The disease most likely arrived in Belgium in the summer of 1845 before quickly spreading to much of Western Europe.[26]

From 150-year-old dried leaves, scientists have now figured out the genome of the single-celled organism that caused the potato blight from 1845 to 1852.[26] It is the first ancient plant to have its DNA decoded.[26] It was found that the sequence was that of the plague-causing bacteria responsible for the Black Death of the 1340s.[27] This Black Death killed millions of Europeans during the 14th century leaving its mark on the human genome, favouring those who carry certain immune system genes and explaining why Europeans respond differently to certain diseases and are more susceptible to autoimmune disorder.[36]

Dr. Jean Ristaino from North Carolina State University has extracted strands of DNA from potato leaves preserved from the Irish Potato Famine from 1845 to 1852.[26] This might answer important questions such as the following: Where did the late blight pathogen, *Phytophthora infestans*, originate?[26] How did it spread to various countries?[26] How has it developed from 1845 to 2013?[26] What are its new genotypes or genetic forms, and how are they different from the old ones?[26] Would this explain the new disease called MS?[26]

Is there a connection between the gene mutation observed in patients with hemochromatosis and the occurrence of the Great Irish Potato Famine?

Before the arrival of the potato disease *Phytophthora infestans* in Ireland, commonly known as blight, the most destructive pathogen to potatoes were oomycetes, a fungus-like eukarocyte.[16] Then in 1868, not long after the end of the Great Irish Potato Famine, Jean-Martin Charcot investigated the curious new disease, later named MS, that was appearing in immigrants of Ireland and the surrounding areas and was able to identify it as a neurological disease.[6] By 1870, American neurologists were also aware of the "new" disease and began diagnosing patients at this time.[6]

Genome analysis of the 13_A2 isolate in individuals with Irish and Northern European ancestry shows extensive genetic breakdown and expression polymorphisms especially in effector genes, where small molecules that bind to a protein can increase or decrease enzyme activity, gene expression, or cell-signaling effector cells.[15,16] Consumption of the potato-blight pathogen, *Phytophthora infestrans*, by Northern Europeans caused changes in the genome that led to amino acid substitutions and resulted in differences in the 13_A2 isolate.[15]

Over 93% of Irish hereditary hemochromatosis (HH) patients are homozygous for the HFE gene with the C282Y mutation, allowing for an accurate diagnostic test of the disease in this population.[4] Mutation in the HLA-H is another candidate for gene screening to determine the presence of hemochromatosis.[18] Although HH is the most common genetic disorder among persons of Northern European descent, hemochromatosis remains relatively unknown.[4]

European-ancestry hereditary hemochromatosis (HH) is tightly linked to mutations within the hemochromatosis (HFE) gene.[4]

In genetic and population studies in Ireland, they indicate how Ireland lost 20% of the population during the Great Irish Potato Famine during the nineteenth century.[20]

Interestingly, multiple sclerosis was one of the topics of study in bioscience and biotechnology from the UK in 1953.[20]

Patients with HH experience excess gastrointestinal absorption of iron, potentially leading to deadly iron deposition in multiple organs.[4] In order to take the necessary precautions for undiagnosed relatives of HH patients, genetic testing of these individuals is often performed so that if they too show the genetic mutations, they can be treated prior to experiencing symptoms and the potentially deadly health problems associated with iron accumulation.[4] Hemochromatosis is particularly predominant among the Irish and other Celtic people.[4]

Does a mutated HH gene play a role in multiple sclerosis?

It was observed that MS patients carrying the mutant C282Y allele for the HFE gene exhibited earlier onset of disease symptoms compared to other genotypes, but it warrants further study in a larger series of MS patients.[4] However, the second HFE gene mutation, H63D, has yet to be determined within the Irish population.[4] Hemochromatosis is a recessive gene inherited from parents who carry 1 or 2 gene mutations.[19] If only one mutated gene is inherited from either parent, they are known as carriers, whereas individuals who inherit two mutated genes experience hemochromatosis.[19] The 3 mutations of the HFE gene known to date are C282Y, H63D, and S65C, and more variations could potentially be identified in the future.[19] Interestingly, research has thought hemochromatosis could be responsible for Parkinson's and Alzheimer's diseases in some people.[19] Compared to individuals without MS, mean serum ferritin in MS patients was high, whereas transferrin saturation and red cell ferritin were on par.[4] Blood-based ferritin testing performed on MS patients showed elevated iron levels in comparison to non-MS control groups over numerous analyses.[4] The highest levels of ferritin were frequent in patients who required bilateral assistance to walk or were confined to a chair and appeared to be related to the severity of the disease.[4] An investigation was made into the relationship of the high serum ferritin values in MS to the HLA-A3 histocompatibility antigen, a marker of the mutated hemochromatosis gene, which is prevalent in MS patients.[7] A statistically significant correlation was not found between serum ferritin levels and the presence of HLA-A3 mutation of the HFE gene.[4]

The HFE gene is located on the short arm of chromosome 6.[10] The protein product combines with the beta-2 microglobulin and the ferritin receptor to regulate the iron absorption via crypt cells in the small intestine.[10] It is likely that the mutation causes the increased iron upsurge by the small intestine crypt cells.[10] The disease is very common in men beyond the age of 40 years old, and its expression is exaserbated by alcoholism, iron-rich diet, and oral and IV iron administration.[10] In women, iron is lost through menstrual blood loss or abnormal hemorrhages, blood donations, pregnancy, lactation, and iron malabsorption and clinical conditions like celiac disease.[10] The diagnosis is made by increased serum ferritin levels and transferrin saturation and stainable iron in hepatocytes, measured by iron in hepatocytes.[10] Patients with hepatic iron overload, same as hereditary hemochromatosis, have no mutation, and homozygous for C282Y mutation do not reveal iron overload.[10] It is administered weekly or twice weekly by phlebotomy of 500 ml with 250 mg iron.[10] To lower levels to normal, phlebotomy is recommended every 3 months and serum ferritin levels should be maintained at levels below 50 ng/ml.[10]

Hemochromatosis gene HFE Cys282Tyr mutation analysis in a cohort of hospitalized Northeast German patients supports the theory of a north-to-south allele prevalence gradient throughout Germany.[8]

Hereditary hemochromatosis is the most common genetic disease where two copies of this gene are present in populations of Northern European ancestry.[8] In population studies in various areas throughout Europe, HFE Cys282Tyr allele showed fluctuating prevalence rates and decreasing frequencies from north to south.[8] However, most of the German prevalence studies covered the central and southern areas of the country.[8]

The present study recruited 709 consecutive patients at the time of their admission to a Northeast German University Hospital Medical Department. DNA sequencing was used to detect HFE Cys282Tyr and His63Asp alleles.[8] Biochemical testing consisting of transferrin saturation rate and concentrations of ferritin, transferrin, and iron were performed in Cys282Tyr homozygous and Cys282Tyr/His63Asp heterozygous, respectively.[8] Results were compared with previous German prevalence studies.[8] Analysis of 709 Caucasian patients resulted in 650 (91.7%) homozygous HFE wild-type carriers, 55 Cys282Tyr/His63Asp compound heterozygous.[8] The HFE Cys282Tyr allele frequency was 4.44% (reference 8). Genetically determined iron overload was elevated in one homozygote.[8] In conclusion, compared to previous hemochromatosis prevalence studies in Germany using blood donors or employees, this study involved hospital patients who had an alleged HFE Cys282Tyr allele frequency of 4.44%[8] and supports the hypothesis of an allele gradient decreasing from north to south within Germany.[8]

As Zamboni stated earlier, a genetic modification in gene coding for iron binding and transporting proteins might be responsible for iron overload.[2]

In hereditary hemochromatosis, there is, in fact, a mutation that substitutes cysteine with tyrosine at amino acid residue 282 (Cys282Tyr) in the alpha 3 domain of the HFE protein[10]. This mutation in the HFE protein in the crypt cells in the intestine leads to an increased number of receptors for iron in the mucosal cells in the duodenal villi.[10] Findings of Spanish patients with the wild genotype at position 282 showed the possibility of other changes in the HFE gene or other places involved in the disease.[11] The high frequency of Cys282Tyr mutation in hereditary hemochromatosis in patients in Spain indicates this is the most common defect related to hereditary hemochromatosis.[11]

A few inborn errors of phenylalanine and tyrosine metabolism have been identified in the literature shown in figure A below.

Tyrosine is used to synthesize other important compounds in the body as shown in figure A below. In the adrenal medulla, tyrosine is used for the synthesis of neurotransmitters and hormones.[9] The first reaction involves tyrosine hydroxylase or monooxygenase, an enzyme that is iron-dependent that hydroxylates tyrosine to 3,4-dihydroxyphenalanine (L-Dopa).[9] Further reactions using L-Dopa yield dopamine, norepinephrine, and epinephrine.[9] L-Dopa is used for painful muscle spasticity in multiple sclerosis.[12]

Epinephrine and the other catacholamines function as hormones in the body and have a huge influence on nutrient metabolism (p. 199).[9]

In the skin, eye, and hair cells in the melanocytes, tyrosine is converted to melanin, a pigment that gives pigment to skin, eyes, and hair (p. 199).[9] In the thyroid gland, tyrosine utilizes iodine to synthesize thyroid hormones (see chapter 13).[9]

There are several inborn errors of metabolism with phenylalanine and tyrosine that have been identified and shown in figure A below. This autosomal recessive genetic disorder occurs with phenylketonuria or PKU.[9] The complication occurs when the enzyme phenylhydroxylase converts phenylalanine to tyrosine.[9] The defect results in an excess of phenylalanine and phenylalanine metabolites (phenylactate, phenylpyruvate, phenylacetate) in the blood and other body fluids.[9]

With the conversion of phenylalanine to tyrosine impaired, blood tyrosine is reduced.[9] If not treated, PKU causes neurological problems such as seizures and hyperactivity[9]. Therefore, it is treated with a phenalanine-restricted diet, and tyrosine must be added to the diet[9].

This can be treated with a phenylalanine-restricted diet.[9] Therefore, protein-containing foods are avoided, and tyrosine must be added to the diet because the body cannot make it.[9]

Another inborn error of metabolism is known as tyrosinemia type 11.[9]

This results in impaired activity of the enzyme aminotransferase that converts tyrosine to p-hydroxyphenylpyruvate.[9]

It is characterized by plasma tyrosine levels, skin and eye lesions, and impaired mental development, which are influenced by nutrient metabolism.[9] People with this problem cannot have phenylalanine or tyrosine.[9]

Another error involving tyrosine degradation is alkaptonuria, resulting from the defective enzyme homogentisate dioxygenase.[9] It normally converts homogentistic acid to maleylacetoacetate and has high levels of homogentistic acid in body tissues and fluids.[9] This acid oxidizes and turns a dark colour, making the urine look black when exposed to air.[9] People with this issue experience arthritis or joint problems from homogentistic acid building up in connective tissues.[9]

LIVER CATABOLISM AND USES OF SULFUR-CONTAINING AMINO ACIDS

The breakdown of methionine, an S-containing essential amino acid (present in the diet) occurs mostly in the liver and produces another S-containing nonessential amino acid (produced in our body), cysteine.[9]

With oxygen, methionine yields succinyl-CoA and is therefore a glucogonic amino acid.[9] In the breakdown of methionine is the conversion of methionine to S-adenosyl methionine (SAM) by methionine adenosyltransferase (in high levels in the liver) in an ATP-involving reaction.[9] SAM assists in further methionine catabolism; it triggers cystathionine synthase that converts homocysteine to cystathionine.[9] SAM also blocks methylenetetrahydrofolate (THF) reductase activity, constituting 5-methyl-THF (also known as N5-methyl-THF) used to change methionine from homocysteine.[9]

When SAM is present in higher levels, it assists the breakdown of methionine, not its repair.[9] SAM is also a main methyl donor and is necessary for synthesis of melatonin, carnitine, creatinine, and epinephrine.[9] It's also required for the metabolism of arsenic.[9] Also, the methyl group from SAM is to methylate DNA and influences gene expression.[9] SAM can be decarboxylated to configure S-adenosyl methylthiopropylamine, involved in the synthesis of the following polyamines important in cell division and growth: spermine, spermidine, and putrescine.[9]

Eliminating or donation of the methyl group from SAM forms S-adenosylhomocysteine (SAH).[9] SAH can be changed to homocysteine

15

by the enzyme S-adenosylhomocysteine hydrolase.[9] Methionine is formed from homocysteine and converted back in a betaine-dependent reaction or vitamin B12 (methylcobalamin) and folate (5-methyl-THF) dependent reaction.[9]

Betaine, produced in the liver from choline oxidation, provides a methyl group that is moved to homocysteine by the hepatic enzyme homocysteine methyltransferase or obtained from the diet.[9]

The loss of the methyl group, betaine is changed to dimethylglycine and further demethylated to produce glycine.[9] In the figure below (6.12, chapter 6), vitamin B12 and folate-dependent methylation reaction, methylcobalamin directly provides the methyl group to remethylate homocysteine to produce methionine.[9] Methylcobalamin picks up the methyl group from 5-methyl-THF.[9] High levels of plasma homocysteine interfere with collagen cross-linking[9] in bone and increase fracture risk, and a risk factor for heart disease may develop if folate, vitamin B12, and/ or vitamin B6 levels are low.[9]

Further degradation, homocysteine forms cystathionine from cystathionine beta synthase.[9] Vitamin B6 in its coenzyme PLP is required for this to happen, and vitamin B6 status to prevent elevated homocysteine levels in the blood.[9]

And further degradation of cystathionine requires a B6-dependent enzyme to produce the amino acid cysteine that produces alpha-ketobutyrate and decarboxylated to propionyl-CoA.[9] The change of homocysteine to cysteine by cystathionine lysase and cystathionine synthase is also called transsulfation pathway.[9] These changes occur in the liver but also in the pancreas, kidney, and intestines.[9]

Alpha-ketobutyrate produces propionyl-CoA, then degraded to D-methylmalonyl-CoA by biotin—dependent enzyme propionyl-CoA carboxylase.[9] D-methylmalonyl-CoA is then degraded to L-methylmalonyl-CoA by a racemase or inversion of asymmetric groups.[9] Finally, vitamin B12—dependent enzyme methylmalonyl-CoA mutase degrades L-methylmalonyl-CoA to the TCA cycle intermediate succinyl-CoA.[9]

DISORDERS OF METHIONINE METABOLISM

From the defective enzyme methionine adenosyltransferase that changes methionine to S-adenosylmethionine (SAM) caused by the genetic disorder hypermethionemia, high blood concentrations of (identified by high blood concentrations of methionine[9]). Therefore a diet should be restricted in methionine but with increased cysteine.[9]

Defects in the enzyme in cystathionine beta synthase that degrades homocysteine to cystathionine cause the genetic disorder homocystinuria.[9] It affects only 1 in 200-300,000 people worldwide but 1 in 65,000 in Ireland.[9] People with this condition show high blood homocysteine and methionine levels and low blood cysteine levels.[9] High plasma homocysteine levels support blood clot or thrombi formation.[9] Other problems include skeletal difficulties, osteoporosis, visual problems, and mental handicaps.[9] For a diet low in methionine and with low intakes of protein foods, added cysteine and possible supplements of betaine and folate are needed.[9]

DISORDERS OF METHIONINE
METABOLISM CONT.

Propionic acidemia is another genetic disorder with an incidence of 1 in 35,000 to 70,000 with 1 in 1,000 in Greenland and 1 in 2-3,000 in Saudi Arabia from errors in the enzyme propionyl-CoA carboxylase, a biotin-dependent enzyme.[9] In the same pathway is the genetic error methylmalonic acidemia, caused by the impaired enzyme[9] methylmalonyl-CoA mutase.[9] It has an incidence of 1 in 48,000. Propionic acidemia is distinguished by accumulation of propionic acid in body fluids,[9] and in methylmalonic academia, the two methylmalonic acids and proprionic acid.[9] Compounds such as methylcitrate, tiglic acid, and 3-hydroxypropionate collect in body fluids. Symptoms in infants are vomiting, low weight, ketoacidosis, hypertonia, and breathing problems as well as other difficulties.[9] Both proprionyl-CoA and methylmalonyl-CoA are degraded from methionine (shown in Figure B) and also from threonine (shown later in Figure 6.15) and isoleucine, and because the breakdown of valine produces methylmalonyl-CoA (shown in Figure 6.36 in chapter 6), the diet requires restriction of various amino acids.[9] As well, odd—chain fatty and polyunsaturated fatty acids in exuberant amounts bring propionyl-CoA and must be restricted.[9]

Biotin supplements have been shown to work with CoA carboxylase, but a restricted diet is still required.[9] Additionally, vitamin B12 supplements can help with the enzyme methylmalonyl-CoA mutase (vitamin B12—dependent) activity in some people with methylmalonic acidemia.[9] A nonessential amino acid can become essential, like tyrosine degraded from essential amino acid phenylalanine.[9] If the diet fails or the body cannot make it as happens in phenylketonuria. PKU is a metabolic genetic disorder in the gene for the hepatic enzyme phenylalanine hydroxylase, necessary to metabolize phenylalanine to tyrosine (see figure A below).[9]

When PKU is untreated, it can lead to mental retardation, seizures, and other serious medical conditions.[9] The medical treatment for PKU is a strict diet, a PHE-restricted diet supplemented with a medical formula with amino acids and other nutrients and maintained for life.[9] Cysteine is a nonessential amino acid used for protein synthesis and used to synthesize homocysteine and also degraded by enzyme cysteine dioxygenase to cysteine sulfinate to produce taurine.[9]

Taurine is made in the liver, is a beta sulfonic acid, and is found in muscle and in the central nervous system[9] and also in less amounts in the heart, kidney, liver, and other tissues.[9] It is not involved in receptors and helping structure and function of photoreceptor cells.[9] It is thought to carry on membrane balance collecting peroxidative products oxychloride.[9]

Taurine also acts as a bile salt in the liver and intestine taurocholate and in the CNS as an inhibitory neurotransmitter.[9]

Finally, cysteine degradation produces pyruvate and sulfate.[9]

Sulfate oxydase (an iron—and molybdenum-dependent enzyme) is changed to sulfate to be excreted in the urine or to synthesize sulfolipids and sulfoproteins.[9]

Aspartate mutation has also been identified in the literature with hereditary hemochromatosis.[11] It is mostly derived from glutamate via aspartate aminotransferase enzyme activity. This amino acid is common in neural tissue and possibly acts as an excitatory neurotransmitter in the CNS.[9]

HISTIDINE

The breakdown of histidine is shown in figure C; it is a gluconeogenic amino acid and is broken down to alpha-ketoglutarate in figure D. It may connect with beta-alanine to produce carnosine.[9]

Read more in chapter 6 in "Advanced Nutrition and Human Metabolism" on nitrogen-containing nonprotein compounds. As well, with a vitamin B6—dependent decarboxylation, histidine is formed from histamine. Histamine works as a neurotransmitter in the brain and stimulates[9] hydrochloric acid in the gastrointestinal tract.[9] Additionally, histamine has immunological roles such as in mast cells located within the nose, mouth, blood vessels, and internal body surfaces and in white blood cells such as basophils.[9] It causes constriction of smooth muscle and dilation or increased permeability of capillaries to aid white blood cells to go through and ingest foreign invaders or antigens by phagocytes.[9]

This may cause redness of skin and escaping of fluid such as a runny nose and watery eyes.[9]

Another interest in the body is its posttranslational modification or biosynthesis in some proteins.[9] Some proteins like actin in muscle become methylated histidine, called 3-methylhistidine; it is released but not reused to make another protein.[9] It is as Zamboni stated earlier: a genetic modification in gene coding for iron binding and transporting proteins might be responsible for iron overload.[2]

In hereditary hemochromatosis, there is, in fact, a mutation that substitutes cysteine to tyrosine at amino acid residue 282 (Cys282Tyr) in the alpha 3 domain of the HFE protein.[9] This mutation in the HFE protein in the crypt cells in the intestine leads to an increased number of receptors for iron in the mucosal cells in the duodenal villi.[10] Findings of Spanish patients with the wild genotype at position 282 showed the possibility of other changes in the HFE gene or other places involved in disease.[11] The high frequency of Cys282Tyr mutation in hereditary hemochromatosis in patients in Spain indicates this is the most common defect related to hereditary hemochromatosis.[11]

In another paper, they indicate people carrying at-risk alleles could be chosen in advance for therapeutic trials for iron chelation and dietary changes due to MS being genetically targeted. Thus, larger studies on iron genes should be a priority in MS[25]. My next discussion is on foods to eat that assist in iron absorption due to iron overload or low iron.

If a person has high levels of iron, consume foods or substances that lower the amount of iron absorbed. People with complicated iron-balance issues will need to work out an individual diet plan starting with a diet for iron balance.[23]

Oxalates are found in spinach, kale, rhubarb, beets, nuts, tea, chocolate, strawberries, wheat bran, and herbs such as oregano, basil, and parsley, impairing the absorption of nonheme iron.[23] The small particles of sand or dirt on the spinach may be the only iron absorbed on the plant.[23]

Oxalates - Non-Heme Iron Inhibitors

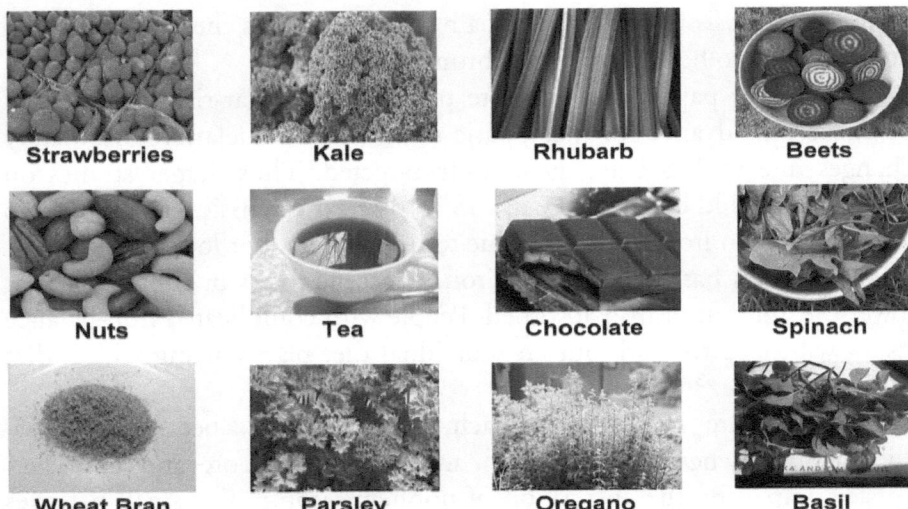

Strawberries   Kale   Rhubarb   Beets

Nuts   Tea   Chocolate   Spinach

Wheat Bran   Parsley   Oregano   Basil

Polyphenols - Non-Heme Iron Inhibitors

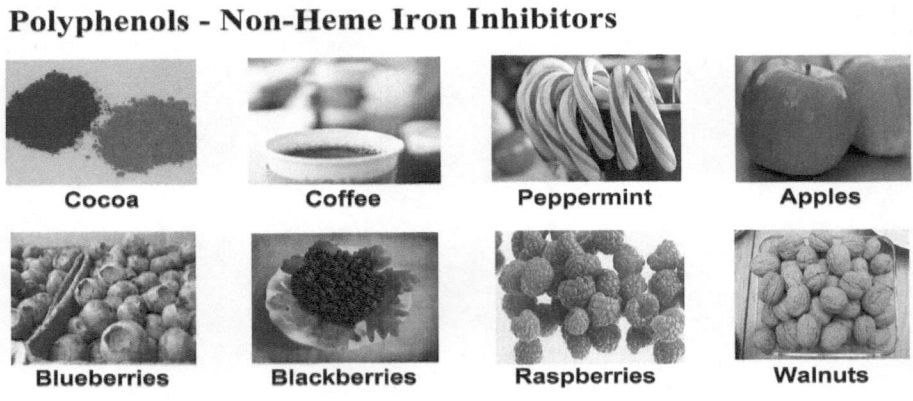

Cocoa   Coffee   Peppermint   Apples

Blueberries   Blackberries   Raspberries   Walnuts

Polyphenols are significant inhibitors of iron absorption found in cocoa, coffee, and various herbs.[23] Also, phenolic compounds inhibit iron absorption found in peppermint, apples, and some herbal teas and tannins found in black tea, coffee, cocoa, walnuts, spices, and fruits such as blueberries, blackberries, and raspberries.[23] Some Swedish teas and cocoa inhibit as much as 90% of iron and 60% in coffee and should not be consumed 2 hours prior to or following a iron-rich meal.[23]

To increase iron absorption, certain foods should be incorporated. One hundred milligrams of Vitamin C enhances the absorption of iron from a specific meal by 4.14 times.[23]

If a person has high levels of iron, consume foods or substances that lower the amount of iron absorbed. People with complicated iron-balance issues will need to work out an individual diet plan, starting with a diet for iron balance.

Calcium - Heme and Non-Heme Iron Inhibitors

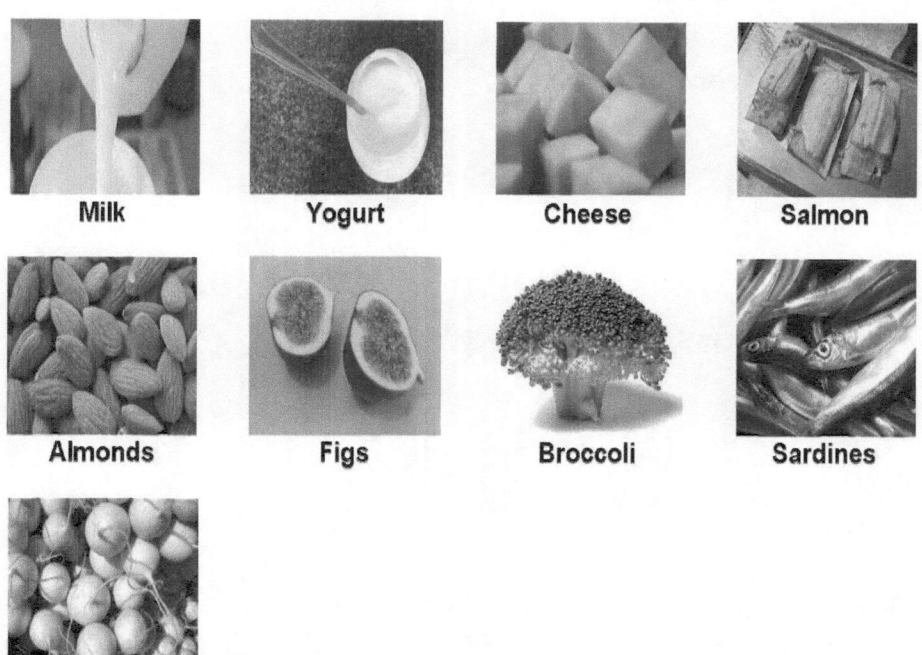

Milk   Yogurt   Cheese   Salmon

Almonds   Figs   Broccoli   Sardines

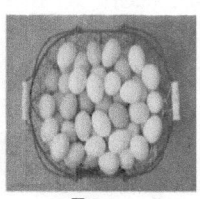

Turnips

Phosvitin - Iron Inhibitor

Eggs

Calcium like iron is an essential mineral and can be obtained from the diet.[23] Found in milk, yogurt, cheese, salmon, almonds, figs, broccoli, sardines, salmons, turnips, greens, and rhubarb, it is the only known substance to inhibit absorption of both heme and noheme iron.[23]

Eggs contain phosvitin, a protein with iron-binding capacity that may have something to do with low bioavailability of iron from eggs.[23] One boiled egg can lose up to 28% of iron absorption in a meal.[23]

Phytates - Iron Inhibitors

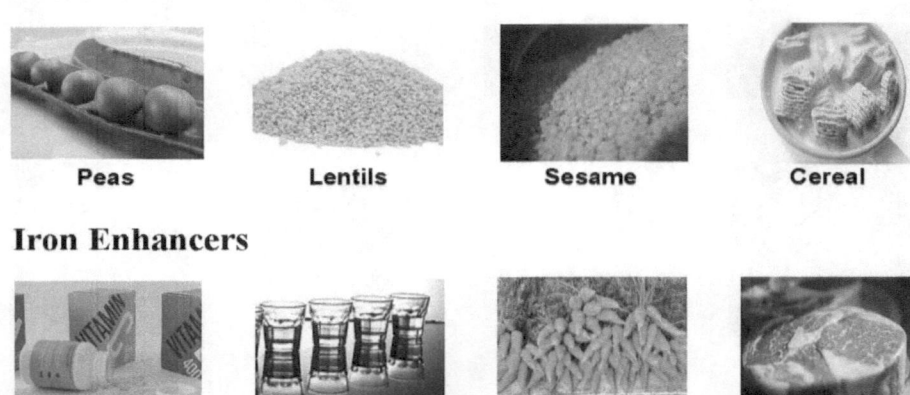

| Peas | Lentils | Sesame | Cereal |

Iron Enhancers

| Vitamin C | Alcohol | Carrots | Red Meat |

Phytates reduce iron absorption by 50-65% and are found in soy protein and fiber and as much as 5% of cereal whole flours have a strong inhibitory effect on iron bioavailability.[23] Phytates are found in walnuts, sesame, almonds, dried beans, peas, lentils, cereals, and whole grains; therefore, you should avoid these if your iron is low.[23]

To increase iron absorption, certain foods should be incorporated. One hundred milligrams of Vitamin C enhances the absorption of iron from a specific meal by 4.14 times.[23]

Although alcohol increases absorption of iron, no one is encouraged to drink. Heavy drinking with high levels of iron increases the risk of liver damage, liver cancer, and red blood cell production. About 20-30% of heavy drinkers get twice the amount of dietary iron as do light drinkers, and if abused, alcohol increases the risk of liver disease such as cirrhosis.[23]

Beta-carotene significantly increases the absorption of iron. With consumption of foods with phytates or tannic acid, beta-carotene aids in the inhibitory effects of both compounds.[23]

Hydrochloric acid (HCI) found in the stomach releases nutrients from foods so they can be absorbed.[23]

Red meat increases the absorption of nonheme iron. Beef, lamb, and venison contain the highest amounts of heme as opposed to pork or chicken, which contains low amounts of heme. One gram of meat has an enhancing effect on nonheme iron absorption similar to that of 1 mg of ascorbic acid.[23]

Refined white sugar has no nutritional value. However, eating fruits or adding honey or molasses to foods such as cereals can boost iron absorption and add nutrients that are not in sugar.[23]

After visiting your doctor and checking for iron overload or low iron levels, your diet should be geared toward iron balance and disease prevention. Iron is distributed throughout the body in hemoglobin, muscles, ferritin, and elsewhere.[23] A healthy diet of fresh fruits, vegetables, adequate protein, whole grains, limited dairy, and fats and sugar will establish adequate iron and lower the risk of disease.[23]

A healthy diet should include the following:[23]

- Fresh fruits and vegetables that include natural hydration and antioxidants.
- Whole grains, which provide fiber and are needed to keep the digestive tract clean.
- Adequate protein, which builds muscle.
- Limit dairy, which causes mucous in the intestines.
- Limit animal fats triggering free radical damage.
- Eat healthy fats found in olive oil and cold-water salmon, avocados, and nuts.
- Limit processed sugars, which contain empty calories and no other nutrients and trigger free-radical damage.
- Whenever possible, consume whole foods. (For MS patients, consider a gluten free diet)

Get at least 20 minutes of physical activity a day.
Note: People with hereditary hemochromatosis should not consume raw shellfish.[23]

RESULTS

In my survey, 70% of MS patients had a Northern European ancestry when asked. However, only parents or grandparents were included. The results may have been greater had great-grandparents been included or known. There may have also been MS patients that were unsure of their heritage due to adoption or it was simply unknown.

Most of the people had ancestry from Ireland, Wales, Scotland, England, Germany, Hungary, Ukraine, Northern France, or Holland.

This is consistent with the spread of the potato blight to these areas in 1845-1852.

In conclusion, the majority of MS subjects are from either Ireland or other Northern European countries where the second mutant gene remains unsolved from the Irish potato famine.

The HFE mutated gene on chromosome 6 combines with beta-2 microglobulin and ferritin that regulates iron absorption by the crypt cells in the small intestine.[10] It is possible that this resulted in a cysteine-tyrosine substitution on the 282 amino acid position.[10] The second HFE gene mutation, H63D, and other unknown HH genes should be investigated further in the Northern European population.[4]

C282Y mutations and H63D mutation in the cis phase might account for questionable ancestry. Iron overload found in MS patients' brains are from a mutated gene found in hemochromatosis in 93% of Irish patients.[4]

Further studies are needed for a thorough screening of the hereditary hemochromatosis, H63D, and further unknown genes of HH in the Northern European population.

TREATMENT

For inborn errors in metabolism, diet management is the only treatment.

Phlebotomy is used as treatment for people with hereditary hemochromatosis to reduce iron stores.[17]

Recently, hepcidin, a key hormone in the homeostasis of iron in the body, is used for the improvement of either iron deficiency or iron overload and controlled by iron stores, hypoxia, inflammation, and red blood cell formation(reference 20).

DISCUSSION

As mentioned earlier P. Infestans genome is a complex genome but much of its Repetitive DNA in comparison to other similar genomes, showed expansion of disease effect or proteins that alter host physiology. [12] A lot of the plant effectors cells have showed effectors to possess cysteine protease or tyrosine phosphotase activity and provided new clues to bacterium-plant interactions.[12]

A ferriscan is a non-invasive,MRI—based diagnostic tool that captures images that provides an accurate measurement of liver iron concentration(LIC).[28] It's used for iron overload such as blood disorders; thalassemia, sickle cell anemia, Diamond Blackfan anemia, myelodysplastic syndrome and hemochromatosis causing a high uptake from the diet.[28]

Look at your ferritin,%Transaturation,measures of albumin! bilirubin! alkaline phosphatase! AFT test (all blood work) CBC like Hgb,platelet count, RDW, and MCV. Methionine is formed from Homocysteine and plasma total homocysteine concentrations reflect non-protein-bound iron in the body.[29] To reiterate, multiple sclerosis may be involved with the following proteins:

Aspartate is common in neural tissue and possibly act as an Excitatory Neurotransmitter in the C.N.S[9]

Cysteine, is a nonessential amino acid used for protein synthesis. Also used to synthesize Glutothionine and also degraded by enzyme cysteine dioxygenase to cysteine sulfinate to produce taurine.[9]

Taurine is made in the liver, a beta sulfonic acid and found in muscle and in the central nervous system.[9]

Taurine is made in the liver, a beta sulfonic acid and found in muscle and in the central nervous system.[9] In fact, taurine may be an amino acid to investigate further as this level is extremely low.

Aspartate is common in neural tissue and possibly acts as an Excitatory neurotransmitter in the C.N.S.[9]

Epinephrine and the other catacholamines function as hormones in the body and have a huge influence on nutrient metabolism.[9]

Tyrosine hydroxylsase or monooxygenase, an enzyme that is iron-dependent that hydroxylates tyrosine to 3, 4 dihydroxyphenalanine (L-Dopa).[9]

Further reactions using L-Dopa yield dopamine, norepinephrine and epinephrine. L-Dopa is used for painful muscle spasticity in multiple influence on nutrient metabolism.[9]

Tyrosine hydroxylsase or monooxygenase, an enzyme that is iron—dependent that hydroxylates Tyrosine to 3, 4 dihydroxyphenalanine (L-Dopa)[9]. Further reactions using L-Dopa yield dopamine, norepinephrine and epinephrine dopa is used for painful muscle spasticity in multiple sclerosis.[9]

"It's a debilitating disease that afflicts a disproportionate share of Canadians—and now London researchers have found a key clue about how multiple sclerosis starts. Iron builds up in the brains of those with multiple sclerosis (MS) from the beginning of the disease. "In suspected MS cases, the very first time they appear in clinic, if they have an abnormally high amount of iron in the frontal cortex of the brain, that's probably a pretty good sign they have MS or some other white matter disease," said Ravi Menon of the Robarts Research Institute. Scientists have long known there's an association between MS and high levels of iron in the brain but they've been unsure if iron was a cause of the disease or just a symptom. Had no spike in iron been found at the start, that would have suggested that it was just an effect of the disease, Menon said. "We wanted to know if the iron deposits happen early in the process, or whether it's something that accumulates with time as the disease 32 progresses," said Menon, who holds a Canada Research Chair in functional magnetic imaging. That iron was found early on leaves open the possibility it's a cause of the disease, he said. Such a finding might excite those who have put their hopes into a "treatment" pioneered by Italian vascular surgeon Paolo Zamboni, who published a study that claimed those with MS had a narrowing of veins that drain blood from the head, a condition he believed caused iron to accumulate in the brain.

His work led desperate patients to seek surgery in which stents were placed in veins to restore the flow of blood. But while Menon found the right vein in MS patients was narrower compared to those without the disease, MS patients with smaller veins had no more iron in their brain than those with wider veins, at least not at an early stage of the disease.

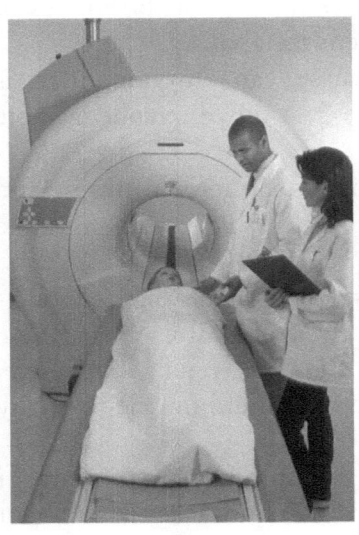
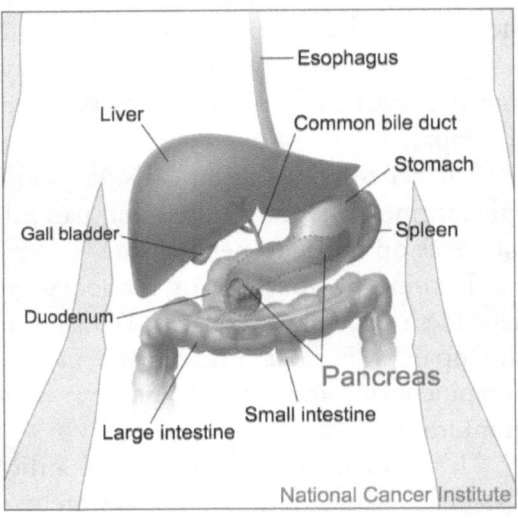

"While the iron in the brain correlates with the disability of the subjects, the iron in the brain does not correlate with the actual diameter of the jugular veins. So the Zamboni hypothesis is incorrect as far as the iron being related to some kind of obstruction," Menon said. The research by Menon and PhD candidate Matthew Quinn was published in Researchers used an MRI to scan 22 patients, at least half of whom will go on to be diagnosed with MS—the others may have a different disease."[30]

Perhaps, in earlier studies a significant interaction was not found with M.S. and Hemochromatosis and serum ferritin because they tested the wrong gene for hemochromatosis. Another interesting fact is the hereditary hemochromatosis with the mutation C282Y and H63D mutations are in the 'cis' phase.[4]

In other studies, sequencing of C282Y and H63D confirmed the sample to substitute lysine for threonine and detected the mutation in cis with G845—> A mutation.[13] This genetic cis formation could be related to multiple sclerosis. Where one side of the body is weaker than the other side.

The results of my blood work tyrosine, cysteine, lysine and threonine were all very low.

The lowest was vitamins B6 used in most enzymes for the previous amino acids. Threonine is only available in the U.S.A. and has been used for the management of spasticity for multiple sclerosis.[13]

Also, I question the enzyme used for tyrosine, tyrosine hydroxylsase or monooxygenase, an enzyme that is iron-dependent below phenylalanine in Figure A.[9]

Ask your doctor to check these amino acids and defective enzymes and vitamins B6 and B12 so you are not deficient or if you are low supplement your diet by going to your local health food store. When checking for hereditary hemochromatosis get genetic testing for mutated genes C282Y, S63C, H63D on the HFE protein in the crypt cells in the intestine which originate from Ireland or other Northern European countries9 and more variations could be identified in the future.[19] The genes C282Y account for 85% and S63C-0.5%and H63D-0.5% does not add up to 100%.

As well, blood tests might not be accurate enough due to hormonal gender differences.

More genetic studies on hemochromatosis, more information about DNA on dried leaves from potato famine from Irish potato famine, and biochemistry on affected amino acids and defective enzymes to follow.

Perhaps the decoded DNA on the 150 year old leaf from the Potato famine and the unknown genes from hereditary hemochromatosis will be provide important insight into the mysterious disease, Multiple Sclerosis.

The great Irish potato famine that occurred in Ireland during the mid nineteenth century has yet to recover from the deaths and emigration that took place. The potato crop had been infested by Phytophthora infestans, an oomycete—a type of single-celled organism related to brown algae which caused the Irish potato blight. The disease most likely arrived in Belgium in the summer of 1845, before quickly spreading much of western Europe. From 150-year-old dried leaves, scientists have now sequenced the genome of the single-celled organism that caused the potato blight from 1845-1852. It is the first ancient plant to have its DNA decoded. It was found that the sequence was that of the plague causing bacteria responsible for the Black Death of the 1340s.[27]

Dr. Jean Ristaino from North Carolina State University has extracted strands of DNA from potato leaves preserved from the Irish Potato Famine from 1845-1852. This might answer important questions such as Where did the late blight disease, Phytophthora infestans originate? How did it spread to various countries? How has it developed from 1845 to 2013? What are its new genotypes, or genetic forms, how are they different from the old ones?" Would this explain the new disease called M.S.[26]

Went to the genetics department at Victoria hospital in London, Ontario, Canada for hereditary hemochromatosis. I was given a sheet of paper with the breakdown of the genes they knew about C282Y-85% S65C-0.5%, H63D-0.5%.

Age group	RDA (IU)	Tolerable Upper Intake (IU)
Infants 0–6 months	400*	1,000
Infants 7–12 months	400*	1,500
Children 1–3 years	600	2,500
Children 4–8 years	600	3,000
Children and Adults 9–70 years	600	4,000
Adults > 70 years	800	4,000
Pregnancy & Lactation	600	4,000

Note*: Adequate Intake rather than Recommended Dietary Allowance.

This needs to be re-evaluated for people with MS.

Recommended Nutrient Intake is Canadian; Recommended Dietary Allowance is American

Written by: Trisha O'Connor B.A.Sc. in Clinical Nutrition

UVB INFORMATION

The active form of vitamin D is synthesized in the skin upon exposure to sunlight. (UVB). It shines on a cholesterol compound in human skin then transformed into vitamin D precursor then absorbed into the blood[36]. It is then converted to the active form of vitamin D over the next day and a half in the liver and kidneys. However, if the liver or kidney is diseased it impairs this conversion of the inactive precursor to the active vitamin and produces symptoms of vitamin D deficiency[36].

Sunscreens with 8 or higher sun protective factors (SPF) can reduce the risk of skin cancer but also prevent Vitamin D synthesis[36].

As well, the pigment of dark skinned people require longer exposure to sun; up to 3 hours for several days depending on climate for several days of vitamin D. Light skinned people need 10-15 minutes to make vitamin D then apply sunscreen[36]. Therefore, people who are housebound from cold climates or intense humidity, such as those with Multiple Sclerosis, or people that work nights or elderly people who unable to get outside or institutionalized end up with a vitamin D deficiency[36]. Vitamin D synthesis cannot penetrate clouds, smoke, smog, heavy clothing, glass or screen windows[36]. Don't be fooled that you are getting plenty of vitamin D on a bright sunny day by sitting close to a window.

Many healthy adults from the north at the end of winter season even those drinking fortified milk with vitamin D, have low blood values of vitamin D[36].

Yogurt and cheese products are often not fortified, therefore reading labels is very important[36].

Vitamin D3 or Calcitriol 1,25-(OH)2 and muscle disorders has been documented with vitamin D deficiency pg. 397 ref. 10. **The common**

problems are muscle weakness and pain, difficulty rising from a sitting position, difficulty walking,especially up stairs, and falling[9].

Biopsies of muscles in individuals with vitamin D deficiency show fast twitch muscle fibers[9]. **These muscles show deterioration of primary type 11 muscle fibers that are used to prevent falls**[9].

Vitamin D supplementation with those deficient increases type 11 muscle fiber and diameter and calmodulin, a cytoskeletal protein, needed for muscle contraction[9].

Calmodulin, in muscle might function through genomic mechanisms to enhance calcium uptake into the cells[9].

Intracellular calcium concentrations are important for contraction and relaxation of muscle[9].

In the early 20th century rickets, a childhood disease characterized by improper bone development, could be prevented by vitamin D in the diet or exposure to ultraviolet light.

Focus was placed on the dietary factor[9].

Calcitriol's target tissues were believed to be in the intestine, bone and kidneys but now known the receptors for the vitamin are found in the heart, muscle,pancreas (beta-cells), brain, skin, colon,prostate breast, hematopoietic system, central nervous system, and immune system[9].

Functions of vitamin D

"Mineralization of bones and teeth (Raises blood calcium and phosphorous by increasing absorption from digestive tract, withdrawing calcium from bones, stimulating retentions by kidneys)"[36]

The active form of vitamin D is synthesized in the skin upon exposure to sunlight (UVB) Vitamin D is converted to 25-hydroxyvitamin D, the major circulating vitamin D and then to 1,25 dihydroxyvitamin D by enzymes in the liver and kidney.[36]

Too little Vitamin D—rickets is a vitamin D deficiency of the bones[36], Children with rickets develop bowed legs because they can't mineralize new bone material, a rubbery protein matrix[36]. Many of these children have a protruding belly from weak abdominal muscles[36].

In the 1700s rickets was thought to be curable with cod-liver oil, rich in vitamin D[36]. Then over a hundred years later, sunlight was linked to prevention and cure of rickets[36].

Today, rickets from bowed legs, knock-knees, beaded ribs, and protruding (pigeon) chests are not common in United States[36]. However, occasionally rickets occurs among breastfed black infants not supplemented with vitamin D, and infants and toddlers fed unfortified beverages instead of formula or milk[36].

Many people around the world suffer from rickets because of inadequate food as well as lack of sunlight[36].

Adolescents who prefer soft drinks over fortified vitamin D milk and prefer video games over outdoor activities during day light hours often lack vitamin D[36].

These teens fail to develop the bone density necessary to prevent bone loss in later life[36].

Older people may be mistaken for arthritis or other problems and suffer painful joints and muscles if their vitamin D levels are low[36].

Osteomalacia is the adult form of rickets and occurs often in women with low calcium intakes and get little sunlight and go through repeated pregnancies and lactation[36]. Given this combination, bone proteins fail to mineralize normally and leg bones may soften[36].

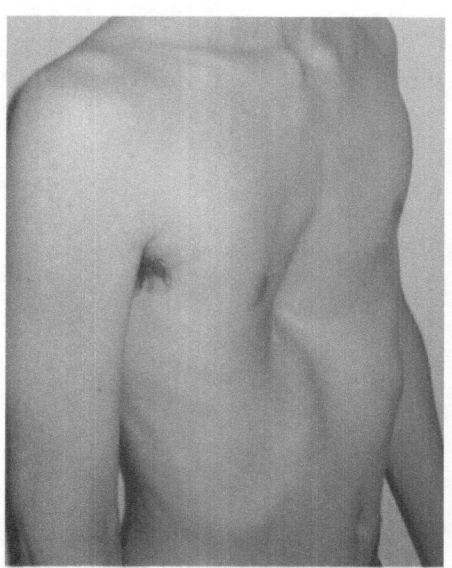

Rickets: a vitamin D deficiency that may
lead to fractures and deformity.

Clinical Nutrition Hereditory Hemachromatosis (HH) and Multiple Sclerosis Symptoms

Hereditory Hemachromatosis (HH)	Common to Both	Multiple Sclerosis (MS)
chronic fatigue	X	fatigue and fatigability
joint pain	X	joint pain
arthritis		
loss of libido or sexual drive	X	loss of libido or sexual drive
impotence	X	impotence
sudden weight loss		
thyroid problems		
mood swings, personality changes	X	mood swings, personality changes
weakness	X	weakness
a change in skin colour	X	
optic neuritis		
spasms		
spasticity		
tremor		
uhthoff's Phenomena (Heat Intolerance)		
irregular heartbeat	X	irregular heartbeat

REFERENCES

1. Valberg et. al. 1989. *Can J Neurol Sci.*
2. Zamboni et. al. Aug. 10, 2012. *BMC Med Genet.* 13:70.
3. Walton, J. C. Sep. 1984. *Arch Pathol Lab Med* (9):755-6.
4. Byrnes, V. 2001. *Genet Test Summer* 5(2):127-30.
5. Kelly, J. 2012. *The Graves Are Walking.* College of Physicians and Surgeons, Columbia University, New York, NY 10032, USA: Henry Holt & Co. Tally CL.
6. Dantas, W. Jan.-Mar. 2001. Peru: *Gastroenterol.*21(1)42-55.
7. Meier, P. et al. 2005. *Clin Lab.* 51(9-10):539-43.
8. Tijdschr Geneeskd, 2003. *Afd. Klinische Chemie.*147(14):652-6
9. Gropper and Smith. 2013. *Advanced Nutrition and Metabolism*, 6th edition.
10. Sanchez, M. J. Nov. 1998. *Hepatol* 29(5):725-8.
11. Internist (Berl). Feb. 2013. 54(2)254, 256-62.
12. Best, L.G., et. al. Jul. 2001. *Clin Genet.* 60(1):68-72.
13. Alfano, James R. and A. Collmer. "Type 111 Secretion System Effector Proteins: Double Agents in Bacterial Disease and Plant Defense." *Annual Review of Pytopathology* (Vol. 42):385-414.
14. Cooke, D. E. L. May 16, 2012 *Nature.*
15. Great_Famine (Ireland). *Wikipedia.*org.
16. Cleve. Apr. 2002. *Clin J Med* 69(4):273
17. *J Med Genet.* Apr. 1997. 34(4)275-8.
18. *www.hemochromatosis.org.*
19. Holland, C. 1999. *Personalized Medicine, Population Genetics and Privacy: An Empirical Study of International Gene Banks.*
20. Zhoa, N., Zhang A. S., Enns, C.A. Jun. 3, 2013. "Iron Regulation by Hepcidin." *J Clin Invest.* 123(6)2337-43.

21. Phllips, M., et. al. Jun. 2000. *Mol Diagn.* 5(2):107-16.
22. *http://www.irondisorders.org/diet.*
23. PKU. *Wikipedia.*
24. Gemmati et. al. 2012. *BMC Medical Genetics* 13:70
25. *http://www.ncsu.edu/news.*
26. *Nature.* May 21, 2013.
27. www.resonancehealth.com/resonance/patient_management_guidelines
28. www.resonancehealth.com/resonance/patient_management_guidelines
29. European Journal of Clinical Nutrition (2007) 61, 1359–1363
30. http://eedition.lfpress.com/epaper/viewer.aspx
31. resonancehealth.com
32. http://www.pbiv.com/images/nature/lbp/liver_diagram.gif
33. Problems with Modern Blood Chemistry—YouTube—by Dr. Bryan Walsh
34. Food Pictures, Liver, FerriScan—Google Images
35. Skibbereen 1847 by Cork artist James Mahony (1810-1879), commissioned by *Illustrated London News,* 1847
36. Frances Sizer and Ellie Whitney (2005) Nutrition Concepts and Controversies (10th edition). Thomson, Wadsworth Inc.
37. Elizabeth Pennis, Science February 3, 2014

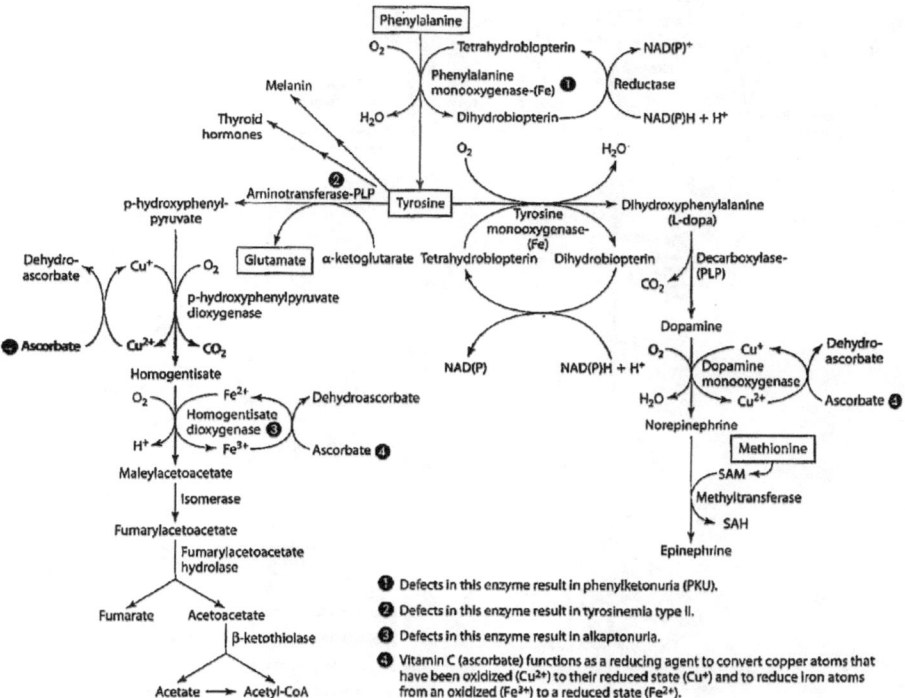

Figure 6.10 Phenylalanine and tyrosine metabolism.[9]

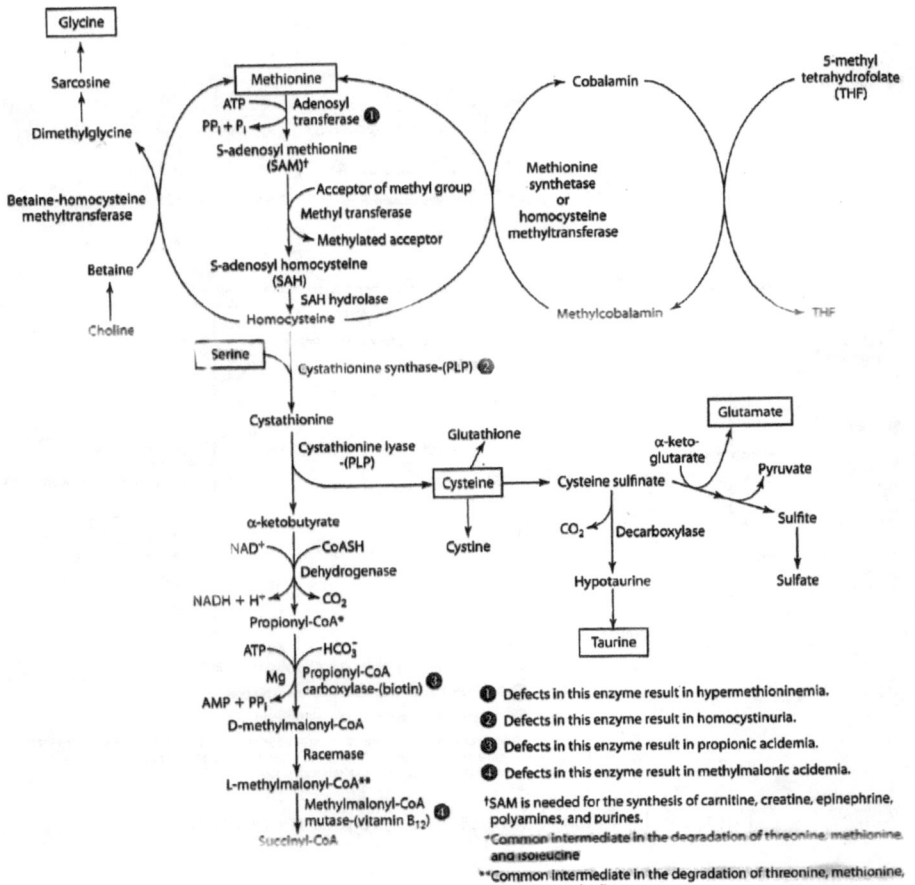

Figure B[9]

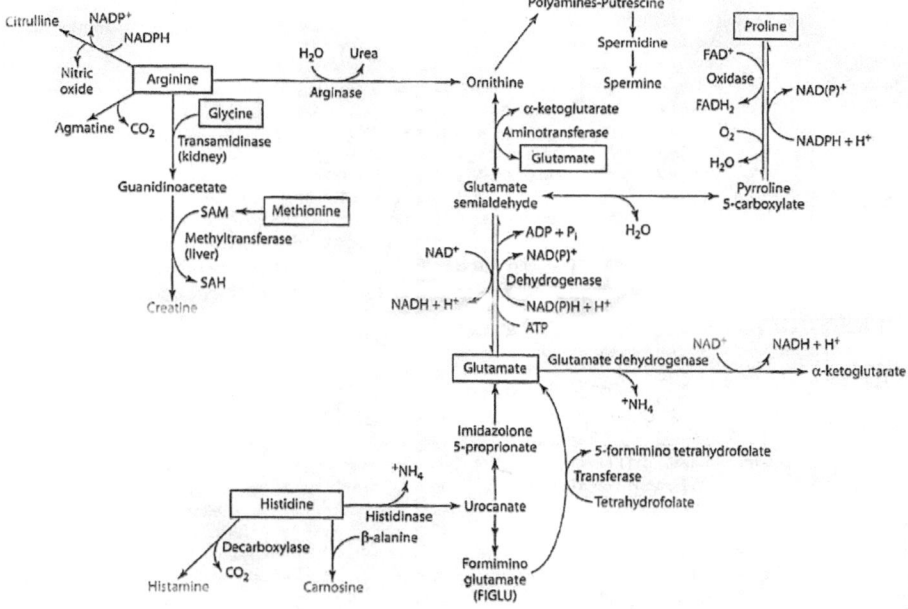

Figure 6.14 Arginine, proline, histidine, and glutamate metabolism.[9]

ATTRIBUTION

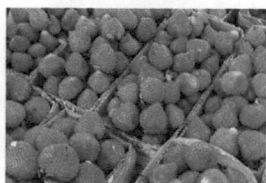

Strawberries
Image: 'Strawberries (La Trinidad, Benguet)'
Credit: Shubert Ciencia/Flickr http://www.flickr.com/
photos/20119750@N00/2404525663
Found on flickrcc.net

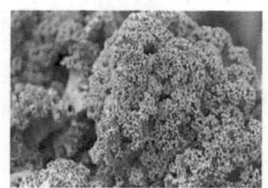

Kale
Image: 'Kale'
Credit: Jennifer/Flickr http://www.flickr.com/
photos/40650893@N04/3923917868
Found on flickrcc.net

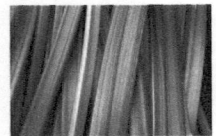

Rhubarb
Image: 'Rhubarb, Borough Market, London, UK.JPG'
Credit: Cory Doctorow/Flickr http://www.flickr.com/
photos/37996580417@N01/2318431953
Found on flickrcc.net

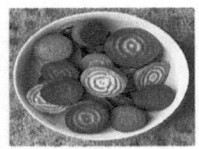

Beets
Image: 'beet bowl'
Credit: woodleywonderworks/Flickr http://www.flickr.com/
photos/73645804@N00/9233914987
Found on flickrcc.net

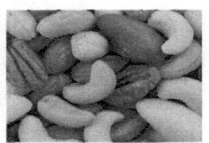

Nuts
Credit: s58y/Flickr
Image: 'STOP & SHOP Deluxe Mixed Nuts' http://www.flickr.com/
photos/45032885@N04/4415406430
Found on flickrcc.net

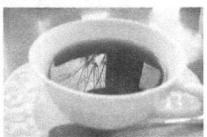

Tea
Image: 'reflection'
Credit: Kanko/Flickr http://www.flickr.com/photos/
29282750@N00/83792141
Found on flickrcc.net

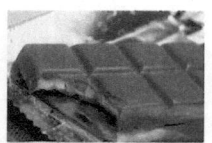

Chocolate
Image: 'Kinder country . . .'
Credit: el7bara/Flickr http://www.flickr.com/photos/
44452545@N00/51886554
Found on flickrcc.net

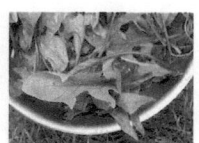

Spinach
Image: 'spinach bowl'
Credit: Ralph Daily/Flickr http://www.flickr.com/
photos/73645804@N00/4633459332
Found on flickrcc.net

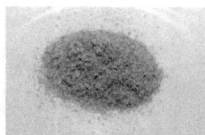

Wheat Bran
Credit: Ali@gwc.org.uk/Wikimedia Commons
http://upload.wikimedia.org/wikipedia/commons/
9/90/WheatBran.jpg

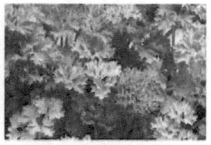

Parsley
Image: 'Balcony starts again II'
Credit: Till Westermayer/Flickr http://www.flickr.com/
photos/98652633@N00/4586500253
Found on flickrcc.net

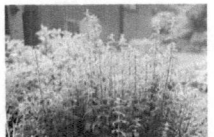

Oregano
Image: 'Oregano'
Credit: Joi Ito/Flickr http://www.flickr.com/photos/
35034362831@N01/2565214027
Found on flickrcc.net

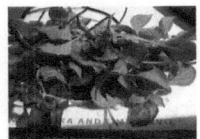

Basil
Image: 'Hydro basil from the indoor garden.'
Credit: Dolen/Flickr http://www.flickr.com/photos/
39804614253@N01/11635085523
Found on flickrcc.net

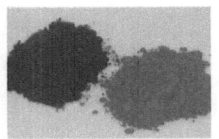

Cocoa
Credit: F_A/Flickr
Image: 'cocoa' http://www.flickr.com/photos/
61404197@N00/5514754116
Found on flickrcc.net

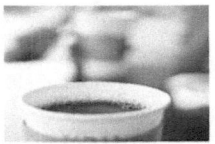

Coffee
Image: 'savor the moment'
Credit: Robert S. Donovan/Flickr http://www.flickr.com/
photos/10687935@N04/3944131005
Found on flickrcc.net

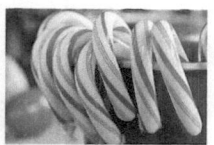

Peppermint
Image: 'Candy Canes'
Credit: Pen Waggener/Flickr http://www.flickr.com/
photos/46286575@N00/6506712013
Found on flickrcc.net

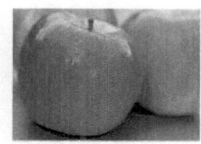

Apples
Image: 'apples'
Credit: liz west/Flickr http://www.flickr.com/photos/
53133240@N00/1517547172
Found on flickrcc.net

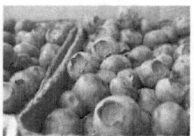

Blueberries
Image: 'blueberries'
Credit: brx0/Flickr http://www.flickr.com/photos/
78153302@N00/257551906
Found on flickrcc.net

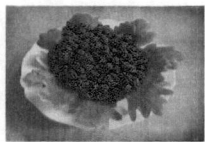

Blackberries
Image: 'Sunday morning pleasures'
Credit: Caroline/Flickr http://www.flickr.com/photos/
20466740@N00/6158084008
Found on flickrcc.net

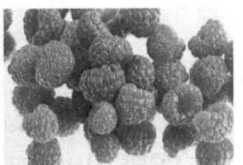

Raspberries
Image: 'raspberries'
Credit: liz west/Flickr http://www.flickr.com/photos/
53133240@N00/3999025000
Found on flickrcc.net

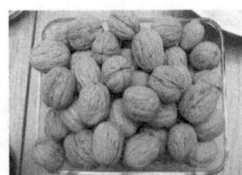

Walnuts
Image: '2010_2107—Food Textures_2'
Credit: Ben Hosking/Flickr http://www.flickr.com/
photos/48004687@N04/4813782068
Found on flickrcc.net

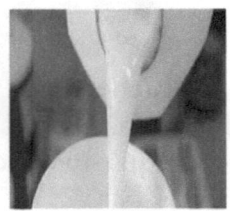

Milk
Image: 'Milk pour'
Credit: Melissa Wiese/Flickr http://www.flickr.com/
photos/93587218@N00/2452046317
Found on flickrcc.net

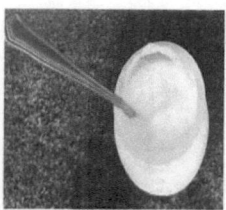

Yogurt
Image: 'yogurt'
Credit: gyroscopio/Flickr http://www.flickr.com/
photos/79253394@N05/7945950036
Found on flickrcc.net

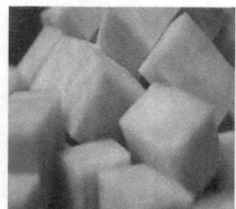

Cheese
Image: 'Cheese 331/365'
Credit: Anne Hornyak/Flickr http://www.flickr.com/
photos/11374291@N05/5766697640
Found on flickrcc.net

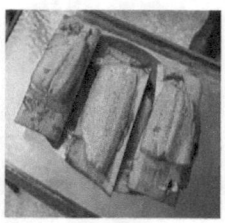

Salmon
Image: 'wild salmon grilled on a cedar plank'
Credit: woodleywonderworks/Flickr http://www.flickr.com/
photos/73645804@N00/822821227
Found on flickrcc.net

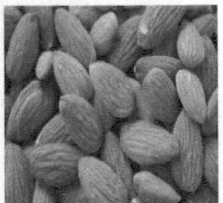

Almonds
Image: 'Almonds!'
Credit: Harsha K R/Flickr http://www.flickr.com/photos/27526538@
N07/3060098365
Found on flickrcc.net

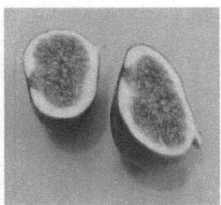

Figs
Image: 'Fig cut in half'
Credit: Richard North/Flickr http://www.flickr.com/
photos/64194289@N04/7960848510
Found on flickrcc.net

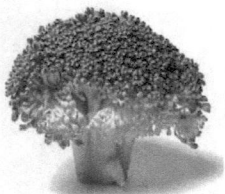

Broccoli
Image: 'Broccolli doesn't grow on trees, you know'
Credit: Darwin Bell/Flickr http://www.flickr.com/
photos/53611153@N00/314088675
Found on flickrcc.net

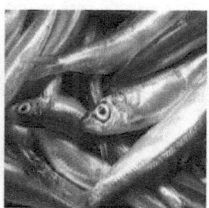

Sardines
Image: 'sardines'
Credit: rockyeda/Flickr http://www.flickr.com/photos/
7774740@N05/600350448
Found on flickrcc.net

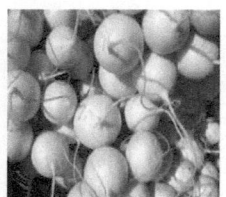

Turnips
Image: 'salad turnips'
Credit: Timothy Vollmer/Flickr http://www.flickr.com/
photos/13102974@N00/2520777271
Found on flickrcc.net

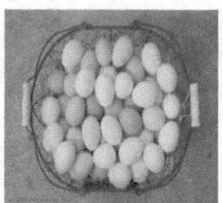

Eggs
Image: 'eggs of many colors'
Credit: woodleywonderworks/Flickr http://www.flickr.com/
photos/73645804@N00/2607036664
Found on flickrcc.net

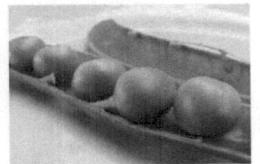

Peas
Image: 'Las perlas de la huerta * Chícharos'
Credit: Jacinta Valero/Flickr http://www.flickr.com/photos/
70626035@N00/8453228965
Found on flickrcc.net

Lentils
Image: 'Red Lentils'
Credit: Rob&Dani/Flickr http://www.flickr.com/photos/
49823770@N00/2889139605
Found on flickrcc.net

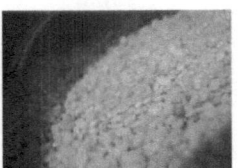

Sesame
Image: 'sesame seeds'
Credit: Nate Steiner/Flickr http://www.flickr.com/
photos/44124484443@N01/27476160
Found on flickrcc.net

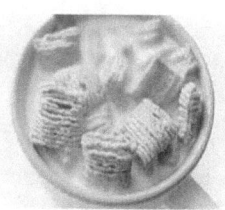

Cereal
Image: 'Wheaties'
Credit: Johnathan Lin/Flickr http://www.flickr.com/
photos/46635911@N00/3599466415
Found on flickrcc.net

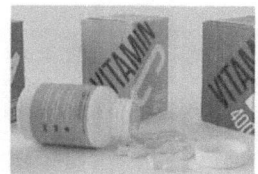

Vitamic C
Image: 'Vitamin Packaging'
Credit: Colin Dunn/Flickr http://www.flickr.com/photos/
31192024@N05/4397922489
Found on flickrcc.net

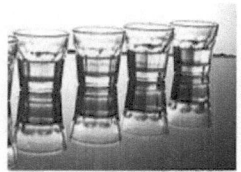

Alcohol
Image: '134/365: Si bebes no conduzcas'
Credit: Andres Nieto Porras/Flickr http://www.flickr.com/
photos/49703021@N00/5718569600
Found on flickrcc.net

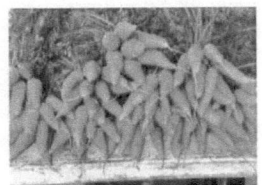

Carrots
Image: 'Farmer's market, Jul 2009—11'
Credit: Ed Yourdon/Flickr http://www.flickr.com/photos/
72098626@N00/3731350661
Found on flickrcc.net

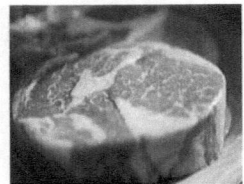

Red Meat
Image: 'Steak'
Credit: Taryn/Flickr http://www.flickr.com/photos/8635903@
N03/6688989961
Found on flickrcc.net

nci-vol-4363-300.jpg (image of a liver is public domain)
Credit: Don Bliss/National Cancer Institute

http://commons.wikimedia.org/wiki/File:Irish_potato_famine_
Bridget_O'Donnel.jpgHYPERLINK "https://overview.mail.yahoo.com?.
src=iOS"

http://upload.wikimedia.org/wikipedia/commons/8/83/Pectus1.jpg